COLD

Hannah O.A

ISBN:9798353430490

DEDICATION
THIS BOOK IS DEDICATED TO EVERYONE TO READ.

CONTENTS

1.Meaning of cold.
2.Types of cold-causes,symptoms etc.
3.How to know when you have a cold.
4.Effects of cold in the body and skin.
5.How to care for your skin during winter.
6.Effects of cold in pregnant women-
causes,symptoms,treatment and prevention.
7.Effects of Cold in babies-
causes,complications,symptoms,treatment and prevention.
8.Effects of cold in children-Symptoms etc.

COLD

What is cold? Cold is the presence of low temperature, especially in the atmosphere. Cold is often a subjective perception. A lower bound to temperature is absolute zero, defined as 0.00k on the kelvin scale, an absolute thermodynamic temperature scale. This corresponds to 273.15c on the Celsius scale,-459.67F on the Fahrenheit scale and 0.00R on the Rankine scale.

Cold can also be defined as:

1.Having a relatively low temperature; having little or no warmth.

2.A feeling of an uncomfortable lack of warmth.

3.Having a temperature lower than the normal temperature of the human body.

4.Lacking in passion, emotion, enthusiasm, ardor etc.dispassionate.

5.Not affectionate, cordial or friendly; unresponsive.

6.Unconscious because of a severe blow, shock etc.

7.Lacking the warmth of life; lifeless.

8.Faint; weak.

9.The relative absence of heat

10.The sensation produced by loss of heat from the body, as by contact with anything having a lower temperature than that of the body.
The opposite of cold are: hot,warm and emotional e.t.c.

Types of cold-causes, symptoms.

1. Common cold/viral cold: it is an upper respiratory infection that is caused by a

virus. Over 200 different viruses can cause the common cold, about 50 percent of common cold is caused by rhinoviruses. When the virus overpowers the immune system and enters the body it causes an infection. It attacks the mucous membrane that is the first line of defense. When this virus enters the cell, it takes control of the cells machinery and manufactures more viruses. This is how we fall prey to a full-fledged viral attack.

Common cold symptoms are:(i)cough(ii)blocked nose(iii)muscle stiffness(iv) breathing difficulties(v)body aches(vi)low- grade fever(vii)post-nasal drip(viii)headache(ix)sneezing (x)watery eyes (xi)sore throat (xii)stuffy nose or nasal congestion etc.

2. Trachea cold/Bacterial tracheitis: it is a collateral damage caused by the common cold. Trachea cold usually affects children and causes a high-pitch sound when they

breathe. It is a sign of underlying serious infection and partial airway obstruction. Staphylococcus aureus bacteria can cause this type of cold. Other bacteria that can cause this type of cold are: streptococcus pneumonia, hemophilic influenza, Moraxella catarrhalis etc.

Symptoms of trachea cold are:(i)runny nose(ii)nasal congestion(iii)repetitive sneezing(iv)wheezing(v)nasal flaring(vi)high fever(vii)deep severe cough etc.

3. Chest cold(lung cold): this cold occurs when the airways of lungs swell and produce mucus in the lungs. This is what makes someone cough uncontrollably. Chest cold is also known as acute bronchitis and last for less than 3 weeks. It is usually caused by a virus and follows an upper respiratory infection.

Symptoms are:(i)mild body aches(ii)sore throat(iii)mild headache(iv)fatigue(v)soreness in the chest(vi)coughing with or with or without mucus etc.

4. Flu: people tend to mistake the flu for a common cold. The symptoms of flu are worse than that of the common cold and people diagnosed with the flu appear to be more ill and experience the onset of chills, fever and headache.
Symptoms:

i.congested or runny nose

ii.a sore throat and a cough

iii.Headaches or body aches.

iv.Chills and shivering.

V.Vomiting, nausea and diarrhea (especially in children).

How to tell when you have a cold?
For example, your nose is running, you've got a cough and your throat is raw. How can

you tell whether you have a cold, allergies or flu?

Cold and flu? Cold symptoms can make you feel bad for a few days, flu symptoms can make you feel quite ill for a few days to a week.

Cold and allergies? This is a question that has been in the mind of a lot of people. Is all that coughing and sneezing from a cold or hay fever?

It is sometimes a tough call but how long your problems last is one of the big clues.

So what are cold and allergies? They have different causes. You get a cold when a tiny living thing called a virus gets into your body. There are hundreds of different types that can make you sick.

Once a cold virus gets inside of you, your immune system, the body's defense against germs, launches a counter-attack. This response brings on the classic symptoms like a cough or stuffed up nose. The viruses that cause cold are contagious. You can pick them up when someone who is infected sneezes, coughs or shake hands with you. After some weeks, your immune system fights the illness and you will stop having symptoms.

It is a different story with allergies. They are caused by an overactive immune system. For some reason, your body mistakes harmless things, such as dust or pollen for germs and mounts an attack on them. When such happens your body releases chemicals such as histamine just as it does when fighting a cold. This can cause a swelling in the passage ways of your nose and you will start sneezing and coughing. Unlike cold, allergies are not contagious though some people may inherit a tendency to get them.

THE EFFECTS OF COLD IN THE BODY.
People may experience:

1.Pain areas in the muscles

2.Cough can be with phlegm (mucus thicker than normal due to illness or irritation, coughed up from the respiratory tract.

3.Nasal: congestion, runny nose, sneezing, loss of smell, redness or post-nasal drip.

4.Whole body: chills, fever, fatigue, malaise or body ache

5.Eyes: watery eyes, itchiness or redness.
6. Head: congestion or sinus pressure.

7.Chest-pressure, headache, swollen lymph nodes (immune system glands that usually enlarge in response to a bacterial or viral infection but sudden swelling of many lymph nodes may indicate cancer). Self-treatment: seeking medical care (consult your medical authority for advice).

EFFECTS OF COLD IN THE SKIN.

Winter, snow, rain, wind and a number of harsh conditions can seriously affect our skin health and appearance. Cold weather causes different reactions on the skin that we need to treat if we want to show a radiant and glowing complexion throughout the whole winter.

Winter skin damage: no matter the number of warm clothes you wear from feet to head. When the temperature drop, your skin moistures drop with them. Your skin gets dry which is the most evident consequence of cold weather on the skin.

While high summer temperatures make your skin produce more oil, cold weather has the opposite effect.

Low temperature are caused by less humidity outdoors and dry environments produced by heating and fires indoors. This temperature fluctuation plus the wind and other outdoor stressors can cause irritation and inflammation. To this, we drink less water in winter. The result is poorer skin hydration e.g. dry, flaky and itchy skin.

Skin micro-circulation is also affected by the cold. Under low temperatures, the skin capillaries constrict in order to reduce the blood flow through the skin. It helps to maintain the body temperature and the capillaries will go back to normal after the exposure. These alternations in skin micro-circulation can cause facial redness, telangiectasia or spider angioma. The effects of the external stressors plus the friction of clothes against the skin can eventually damage the hydrolipidic barrier. Hydrolipidic barrier is also known as the acid mantle, it is a layer made up of naturally occurring oils and lipids that are necessary to maintain skin balance and protect it from external stressors.

HOW TO CARE FOR YOUR SKIN DURING WINTER.

Here are some tips on how to minimize the effects of winter on the skin and prevent dryness that comes with it:

1. Use a skin cleanser: try to use a soft skin cleanser with milder surfactants and fewer fragrances to help to preserve the hydrolipidic barrier that gets thinner and more fragile in winter. Cleanse your hands often with hand sanitizer. To reduce the drying effects of alcohol-based sanitizers, moisturize your hands more often.

2. Avoid too hot showers: Too much hot shower is not good for your skin. Hot water damages the acid mantle and weakens the skin barrier.it can lead to dry skin. Lukewarm water showers are much more advisable.

3. Reinforce your skin moisture in your skin moisture. Use a thicker day cream in winter, add a moisturizing serum to your regime or apply a moisturizing mask more often. You can also moisturize your slip frequently and drink plenty of water.

4. Humidify the environment: use a humidifier at home to counteract the air dryness caused by heating devices. It will make the atmosphere more bearable for your skin.

EFFECTS OF COLD IN PREGNANT WOMEN. According to research, maternal cold or flu with fever during pregnancy maybe linked to birth defects. A study from the Centers For Disease Control And Prevention (CDC) found out that women who had a cold or flu with fever just before or during early pregnancy may be more likely to have a baby born with a birth defect.

Having a cold or flu with fever just before or during early pregnancy can be related to these birth defects:

i.Anencephaly

ii.Encephalocele

iii.Colonic atresia/stenosis

iv.Spina bifida

v.Cleft clip with or without cleft palate

vi.Gastroschisis

vii.Limb reduction defects etc.

Women who are planning a

pregnancy should always protect themselves from fever and infection during early pregnancy to help prevent birth defects.

Birth defects are structural changes present at birth that can affect almost any part or parts of the body (such as the heart, brain, face, arms and legs). They may affect how the body looks, works or both. Catching a cold during pregnancy will not harm the fetus, but it can be uncomfortable for the person who is pregnant and they may also worry about which treatments and medications they can use safely. Colds are very common. The CDC estimate that adults have an average of 2-3 colds per year. According to MARCH OF DIMES, catching a cold will not harm a developing fetus and the pregnant person will typically recover in a week or so. They are also likely to catch more serious infections such as the flu during pregnancy. This means that taking steps to prevent illness is important during pregnancy.

-Pregnancy rhinitis occurs in around 20% of people. Some people may find it difficult to distinguish rhinitis from a common cold.
The symptoms of pregnancy rhinitis include:

i.A runny nose.

ii.Congestion

iii.Sneezing

iv.Difficulty in breathing

v.Snoring etc.

Treatment: The Food and Drug Administration (FDA) recommend always talking to a doctor before using any pain medication during pregnancy.

Prevention: they are more likely to catch colds and the flu during pregnancy. So it is important to take steps to prevent illness.

To prevent the common cold, the CDC recommend:

1.Washing the hands often with soap and water for 20 seconds, or using an alcohol based hand sanitizer when soap or water is not available.

2.Avoid touching the face with unwashed hands because viruses that cause colds can enter the body through the eyes, nose and mouth.

 3.Staying away from people who are sick as close contact with others can spread cold viruses.

Do some moderate pregnancy-safe exercises, such as swimming and indoor cycling can boost the immune system and increase metabolism. Healthful eating is another important factor in preventing a cold. Focusing on eating a variety of fresh foods can help ensure the body gets the nutrients it needs. Taking a prenatal vitamin that includes zinc and vitamin C may also help support the immune system and prevent colds.

  CDC'S National Center on Birth Defects and Developmental Disabilities (NCBDD) saves babies by preventing birth defects. They identify causes of birth defects, finds opportunities to prevent them and improves the health of those living with birth defects.

EFFECTS OF COLD IN BABIES

The common cold in babies is caused by viruses or germs that infect the nose, throat and sinuses. Babies have not yet built up their immune system to fight all of those germs. Cold germs spread easily. Your baby's immune system will need time to mature. Babies do touch things that have germs on them such as their eyes, nose and mouths. They also put things, such as toys in their mouths and touch other babies while they are playing. Cold viruses can live on objects for several hours and can be picked up on the hands of other babies who touch the same object. Some cold viruses can be spread through the air when a sick baby coughs or sneezes. Droplets carrying cold germs from the cough or sneeze may reach another baby's nose or mouth. If a baby touches something that has cold germs on it, then touches his or her mouth, eyes, or nose the germs can infect the baby. Parents/caregivers who regularly pick up a child, change a diaper and feed the baby can also pick up the cold virus and pass the germs to the baby. Babies can catch eight or more during their first year alone, especially if they are in day care or have siblings who bring home germs from school. These sniffles and sneezes in babies are rarely serious, they are tough on parents and one of the biggest reasons for pedestrian visits. When you know how to help your child feel better and when to call the doctor, you can feel more confident until the cold is over. Babies often pick up colds at day care or they can catch it from older brothers and sisters/younger siblings who bring the virus home from school or from grown-ups who shook hands with someone who should have stayed home from work. Babies start to show signs of a cold about 1 to 3 days after they are infected.

Symptoms in young children can include:

i.Stuffy nose

ii.Runny nose, which should be clear at first but may turn yellow or green.

iii.Sneezing.

iv.Fussiness

v.Cough

vi.Fatigue

vii.Trouble sleeping

Viii.Reduced appetite

ix.Fever

x.Vomiting, diarrhea.
Treatment: cold do not need to be treated. They go away on their own after a few days, your child should start to feel better in about 7 to 10 days. Antibiotics can't work because they kill bacteria and in this case viruses are to be blamed.
You will want to stop your baby's symptoms. But don't give over- the-counter cough and cold medicines to infants and toddlers. These products don't work well in kids under 6 years and they can cause dangerous side effects in young children. The FDA advises against using them at all in children younger than 4.

To stop a fever and make your child more comfortable, you can use acetaminophen (children's Tylenol) or ibuprofen (children's motrin or advil) If they are over 6 months old. You can also visit a licensed doctor for more help. Read the package to make sure you give the right dose for their weight and age.

According to the research I did, it is advisable not to give your child any medicine that contains aspirin. It can raise the risk for a rare but serious disease called Reye's syndrome. To help your little one feel better let them have a lot of rest and try any of these home remedies:

1.Extra fluids: nurse your infant more often or give them pedialyte. Babies over 6 months can be given water and 100% fruit juice to them. The added fluid will prevent dehydration and keep your child's nose and mouth moist.

2.Turn on a humidifier: a cool mist humidifier will add moisture to the air and keep your baby's nose from drying out. Wash out the machine after each use to prevent bacteria and mold build up. If your child has croup, inhaling warm steam in the bathroom or exposure to cool air may help with the barky cough symptoms.

3.Spray saline and suck out mucus: if your baby has trouble breathing through a stuffed nose, spray a few drops of a saline (salt water)solution(commonly available in pharmacies)into each nostril to loosen the mucus. Then use a bulb syringe to remove the mucus. Squeeze the bulb and then place the tip into your child's nostril. Release the bulb to gently suction out the mucus. Wash the tip of the syringe with soap and water after each use. If you make your own saline solution, use distilled water or boiled water.

Complications: these conditions can occur

along with a common cold:

1. Acute ear infection (otitis media): this is the most common complication of the common cold. Ear infections occur when bacteria or viruses enter the space behind the eardrum.

2. Wheezing: a cold can trigger wheezing, even if your child doesn't have asthma. If your child does have asthma, a cold can make it worse.

3. Acute sinusitis: a common cold that doesn't resolve may lead to an infection within the sinuses (sinusitis).

4. Other infections: a common cold can lead to other infections, including pneumonia, bronchiolitis and croup. Such infections need to be treated by a doctor.

Prevention; the best defense against the common cold is precautions and frequent hand washing.

1. Wash your hands before feeding or touching your baby: wash your hands

thoroughly and often with soap and water for at least 20 seconds. If soap and water aren't available, use an alcohol-based hand sanitizer that contains at least 60% alcohol. Teach your older children the importance of hand washing. Avoid touching your eyes, nose and mouth with unwashed hands.

2. Keep your baby away from anyone who is sick: if you have a new born, don't allow visits from anyone who is sick. If possible, avoid public transportation and public gatherings with your new born.

3. Teach everyone in the household to cough or sneeze into a tissue: throw away used tissues right away and then wash your hands thoroughly. If you can't reach a tissue in time, cough or sneeze into your elbow. Then wash your hands.

4. Clean your baby's toys and pacifiers often: clean frequently touched surfaces. This is very important if someone in your family or baby's playmate has a cold.

5. Look for a child care setting with good hygiene practices and clear policies about keeping sick children at home.
Simple preventive measures can help keep the common cold at ease.

If your baby has a cold with no complications, it should resolve within 10 to 14 days. Most colds are simply a nuisance. But it's important to take your baby's signs and symptoms seriously. If symptoms don't improve or if they worsen, it is time to talk to your doctor.
If your baby is younger than 3 months of age, call the doctor: in newborns, it is especially important to make sure that a more serious illness isn't present, especially if your baby has a fever.

THE EFFECTS OF COLD IN CHILDREN.
More than 200 different viruses can cause this infection, but the rhinovirus is the most common culprit. Antibiotics which fight bacteria, won't treat your child's cold because a cold is a viral illness. Viral illness cannot be treated with antibiotics. Except in newborns or in immuno-compromised children, colds in healthy children aren't dangerous. They usually go away in 4 to 10 days. Children can be infected with cold when they come in contact with virus-infected droplets of saliva or mucus in the air when someone infected coughs, sneezes or talks or when they have direct contact with an infected person or by touching contaminated objects such as toys. Cold in children starts with a scratchy tickle feeling in the throat.

Other symptoms of cold in the body include:

1.Stuffy or runny nose

2.Chills, weakness or tiredness

3.Sore or dry throat

4. Headaches

5. Mild fever

6.chest congestion

7.muscle ache

8. loss of voice and loss of appetite

9.watery mucus in the nose

10.watery or crusty eyes

11.sneezing

12.feeling of tiredness

13.Fever (sometimes).

14. Throat

15 .Cough

16.Decreased or no appetite.

A cold virus can affect your child's sinuses, throat, bronchial tubes and ears. They may also have diarrhea and vomiting. At first your child may be irritable and complain of a headache and feeling stuffed up. After a while, the mucus coming out of their nose may turn darker and thicker.

HOW MANY COLDS WILL MY CHILD GET? Babies and toddlers often have 8 to 10 colds a year before they turn 2 years old. Kids who are preschool age have around 9 colds a year, while kindergarteners can have 12 a year. Adolescents and adults get about 2 to 4 a year. Cold season's runs from September until March or April, so children usually get sick most often during these months. There is no medication for the common cold. Medical experts say the common cold is a self-limiting illness. That is, it will resolve with time and management. The virus dies off naturally as the immune system fights off the infection. However, medical treatments can be taken to alleviate the symptoms associated with the cold. If an infected child doesn't recover within a week, there's a need for prompt medical attention rather than ignorantly administering antibiotics in various forms. If the cold puts your child in a weak state and makes them vulnerable to other infections, urgently take the child to see a doctor or consult a health worker around you. Use drugs only as prescribed.

Prevention: As a parent, guardian or caregiver, you should keep the infected child hydrated; let them drink plenty of water and warm liquids. You may need to use a humidifier to help ease nasal congestion before feeding the child and to also help them sleep better at night. To shorten the cold duration and avoid complications, allow the child to rest adequately and give them fruits and vitamin supplements prescribed by the doctor. More so, help the child maintain basic body hygiene by making sure their hands are washed regularly. Ensure their nails are trimmed; keep them away from sick people; remind them to avoid touching their eyes, nose and mouth. They should also wear clothes that are suitable for cold weather. Keep the environment clean; use disinfectants to clean up your kitchen, bathroom, toilet and floor. Also, teach your children to sneeze into their bent elbow; they can even make it a habit to cough or sneeze into a tissue paper and immediately discard it.

@CHRISTIAN WOMEN MIRROR (THE MAGAZINE THAT BUILDS GODLY WOMEN). This magazine is not only meant for women to read it is for all gender. The book contains scriptural words, healthy tips, food and fruit and how to take care of your children.

Are cold medicines safe for kids? The FDA (Food and drug administration) and drug makers say you shouldn't give over-the-counter cough and cold medicines to children under 4. These include things like:

1.Cough suppressants (dextromethorphan or DM).

2.Cough expectorants (guaifenesin).

3. Decongestants (pseudoephedrine and phenylephrine).

4. Antihistamines (such as brompheniramine, chlorpheniramine maleate, diphenhydramine and others).

These drugs are the active ingredients in many brands of kids' cold and cough medicines. Children should not be using cough medicines. Coughing is the body's natural way of helping the body to get rid of the cold virus. It is okay to let your child cough, unless they are in distress.

Talk to your doctor if your child did not get better in few days. Also if they have a high fever, vomiting, chills and shakes, a hacking cough, any respiratory distress or extreme fatigue. These may be signs of something more severe, like the flu or a bacterial infection. If your child also have asthma, diabetes or other long term health conditions you can call your doctor to talk about medicine or other treatment.

ABOUT THE AUTHOR

Hannah O.A is a young female writer.She has written a lot of books e.g The family"love in the home"e.t.c.